This book belongs to:

____
NAME:

____
PHONE:

____
EMAIL:

____
ADDRESS:

THE PROPER WAY TO WASH YOUR HANDS

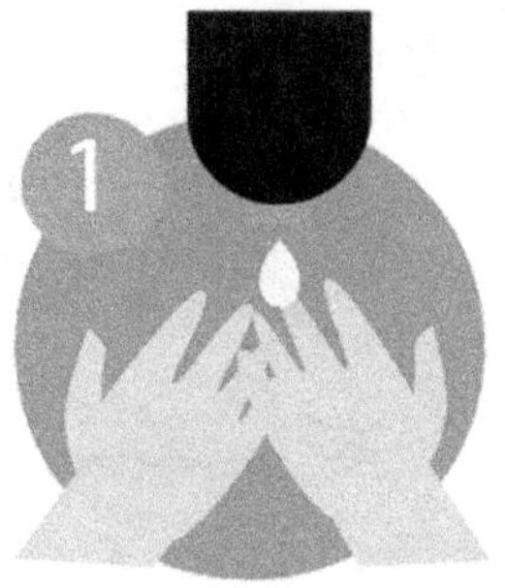

Apply soap
on wet hands

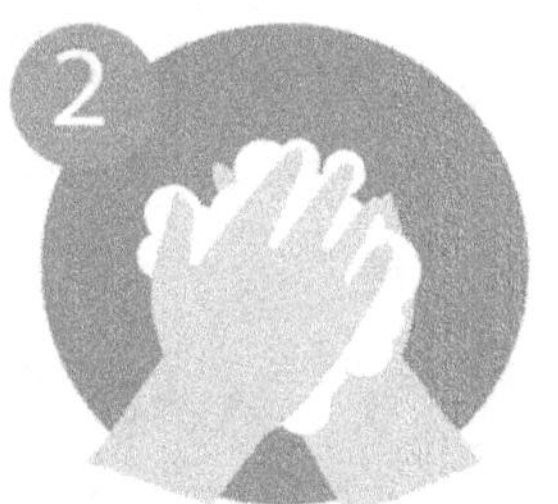

Rub palm
to palm

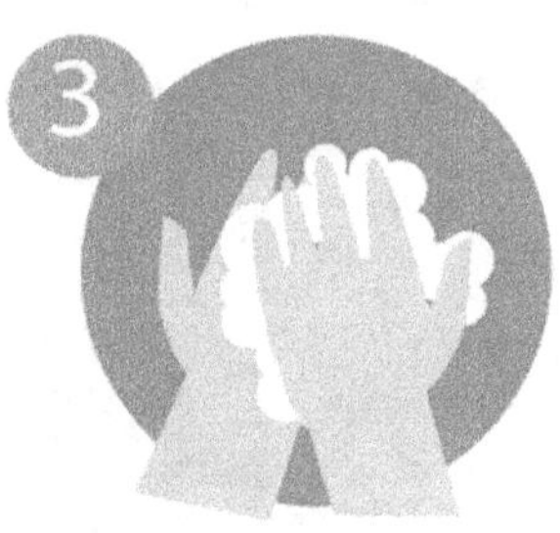

Now, focus on
the back of
your hands

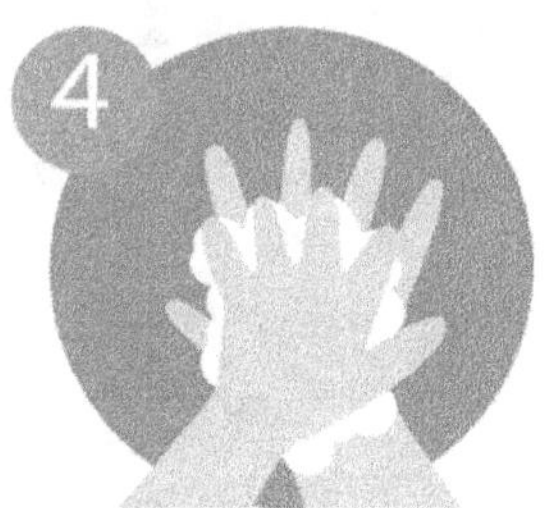

Interlace
your fingers

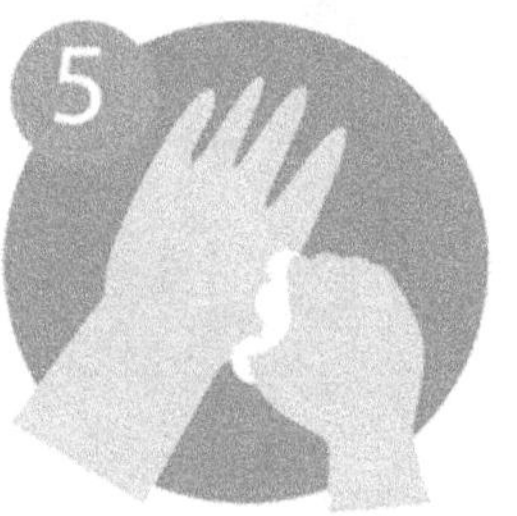

Clean thumbs

Rub nails and
fingertips against
your palms

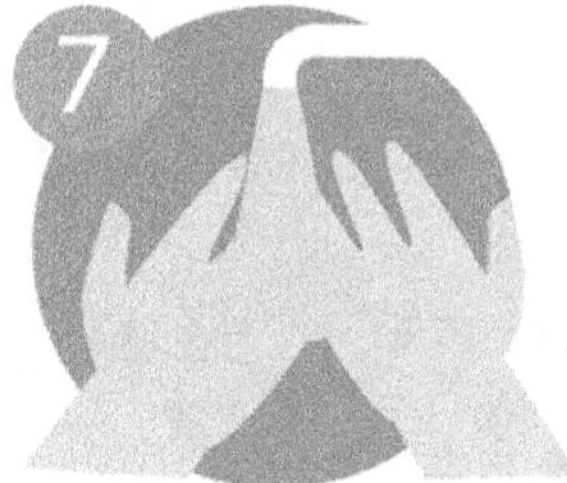

Rinse
your hands

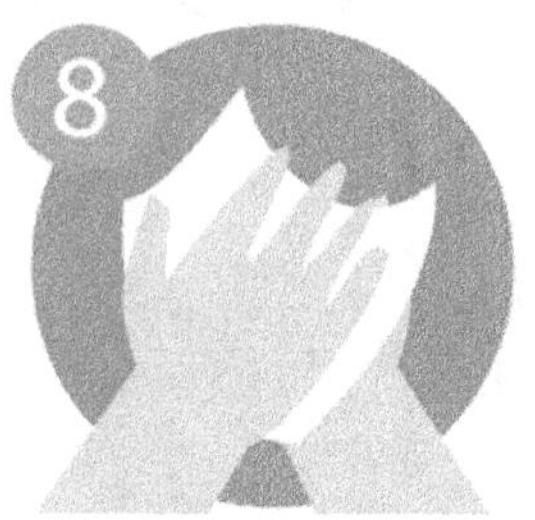

Dry with a
paper tower

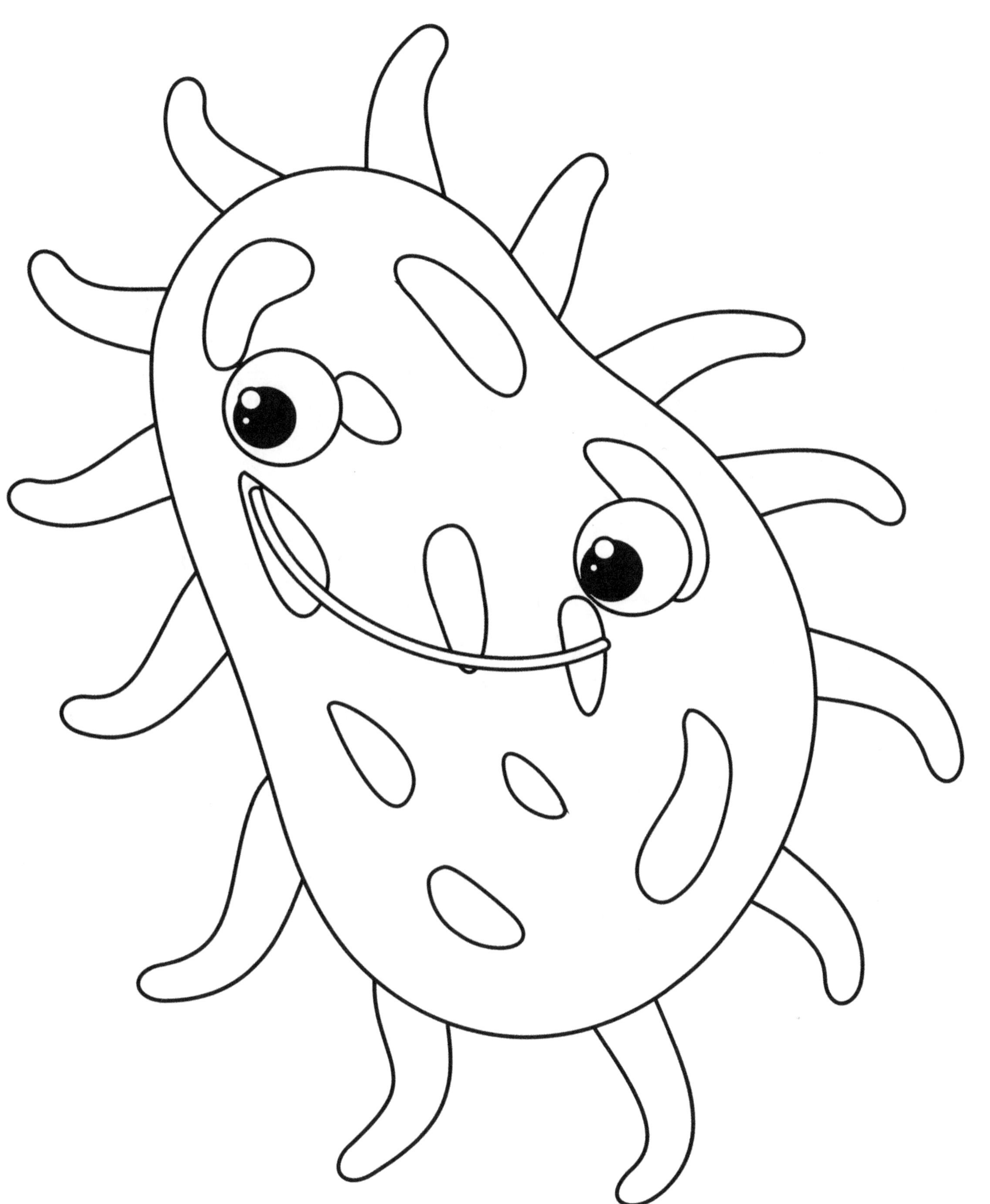

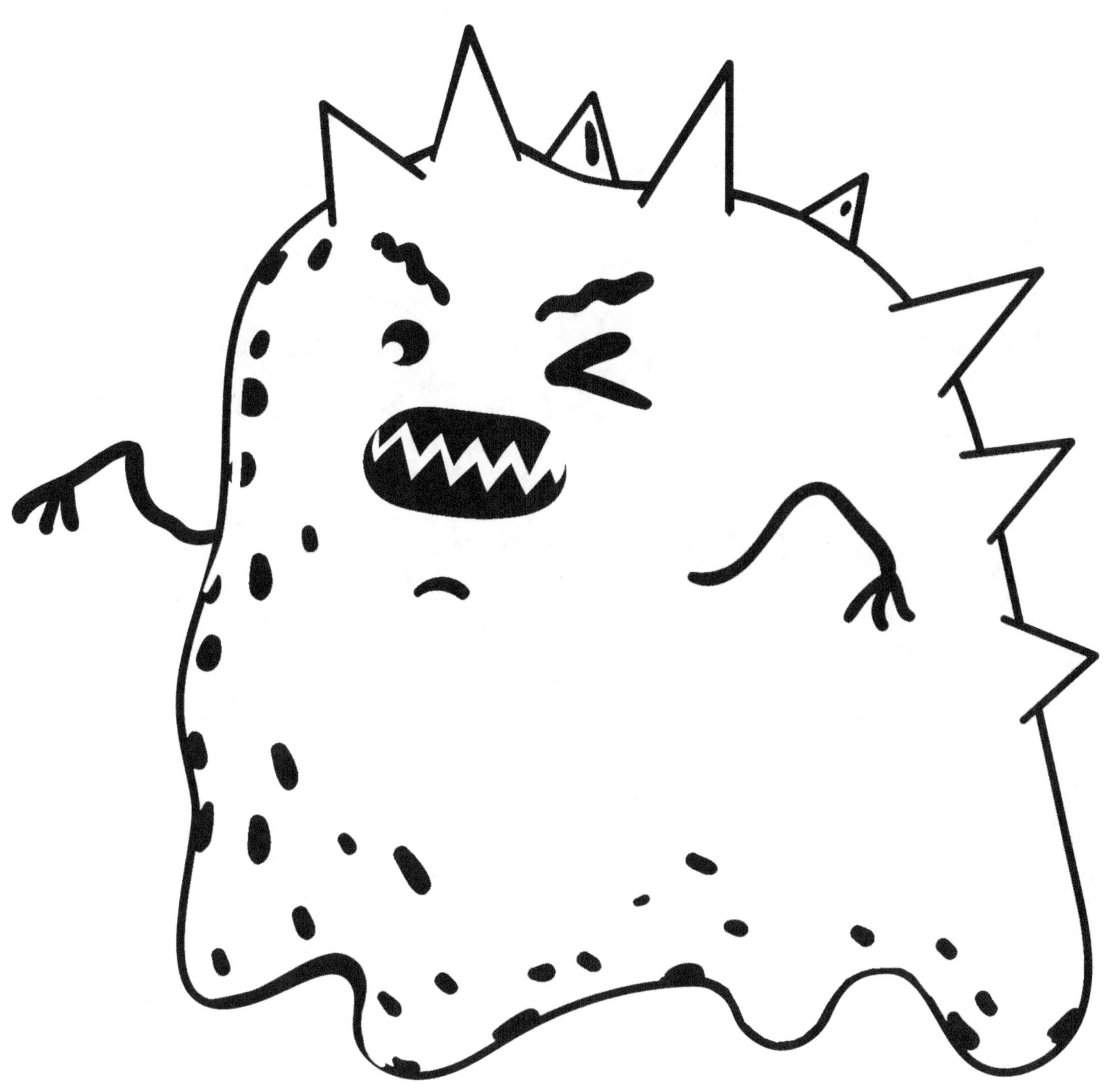

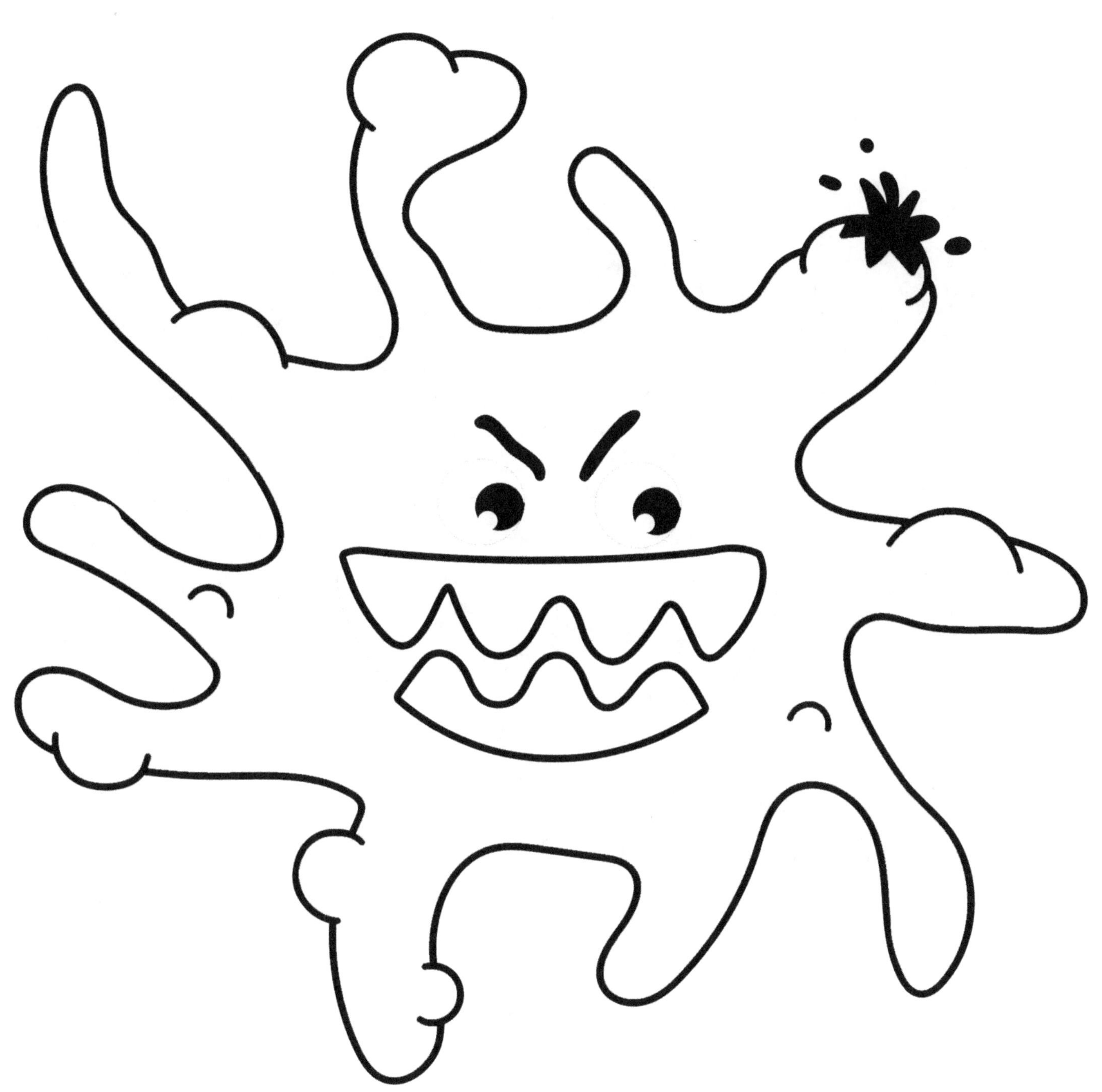

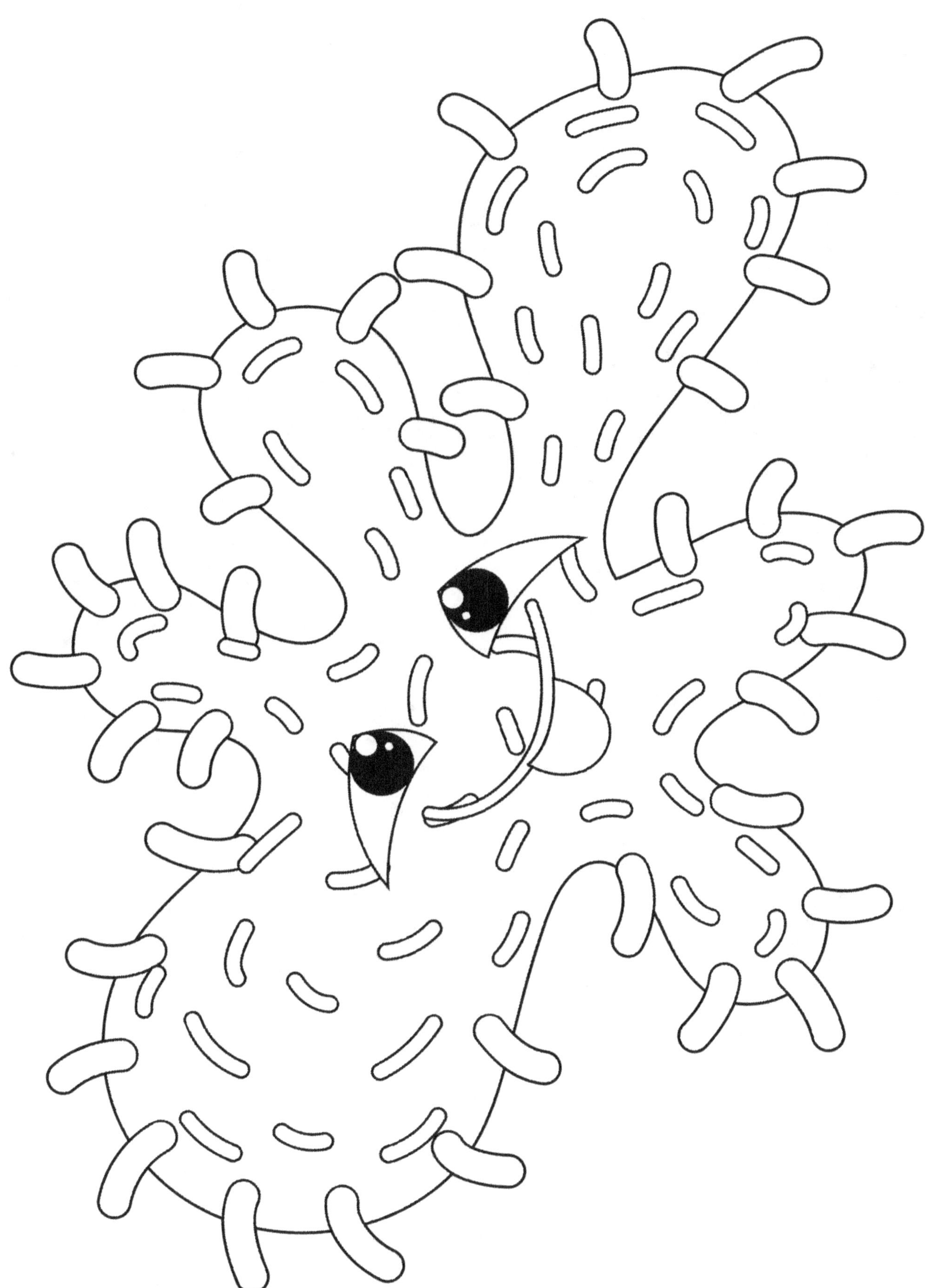

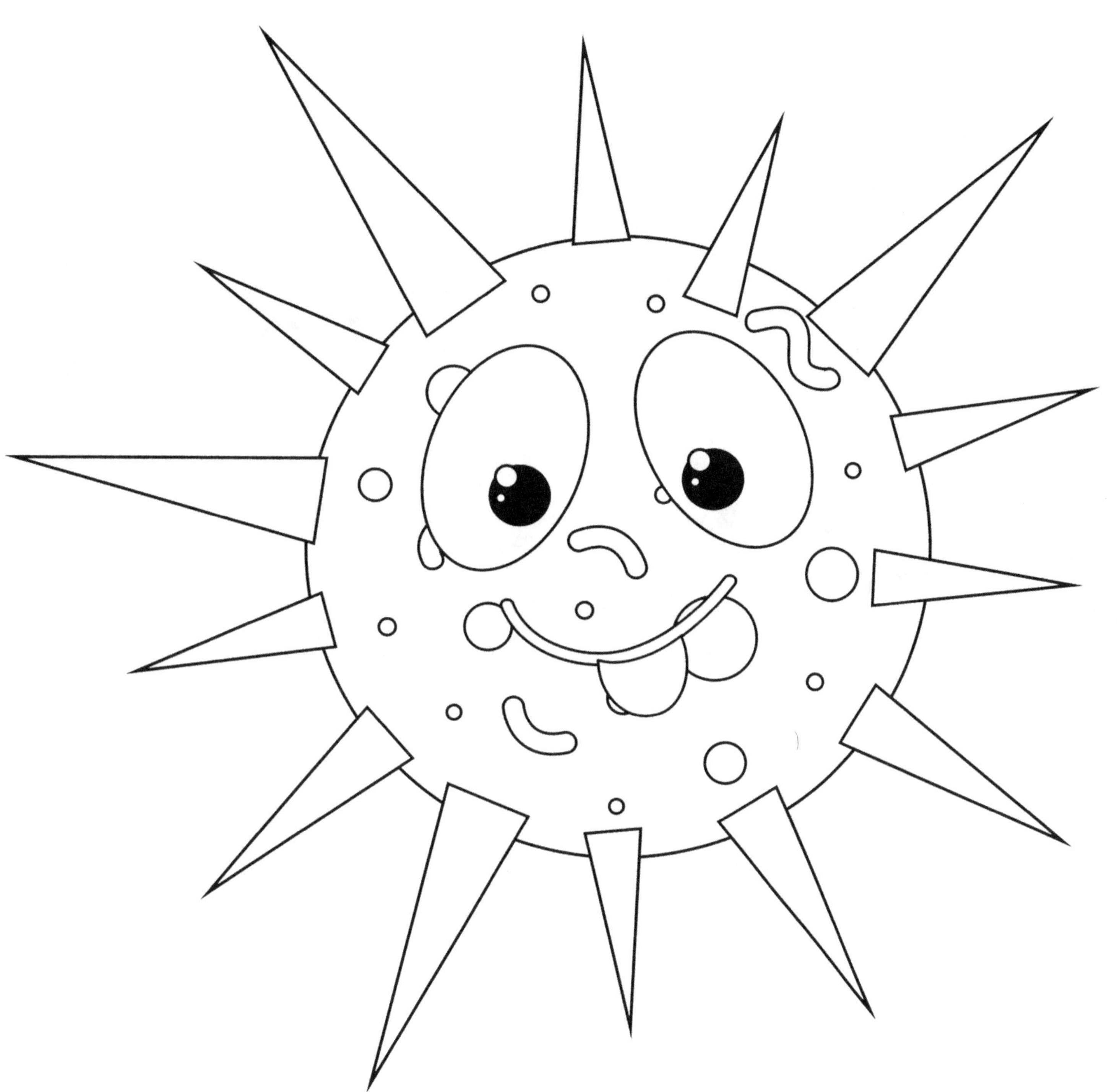

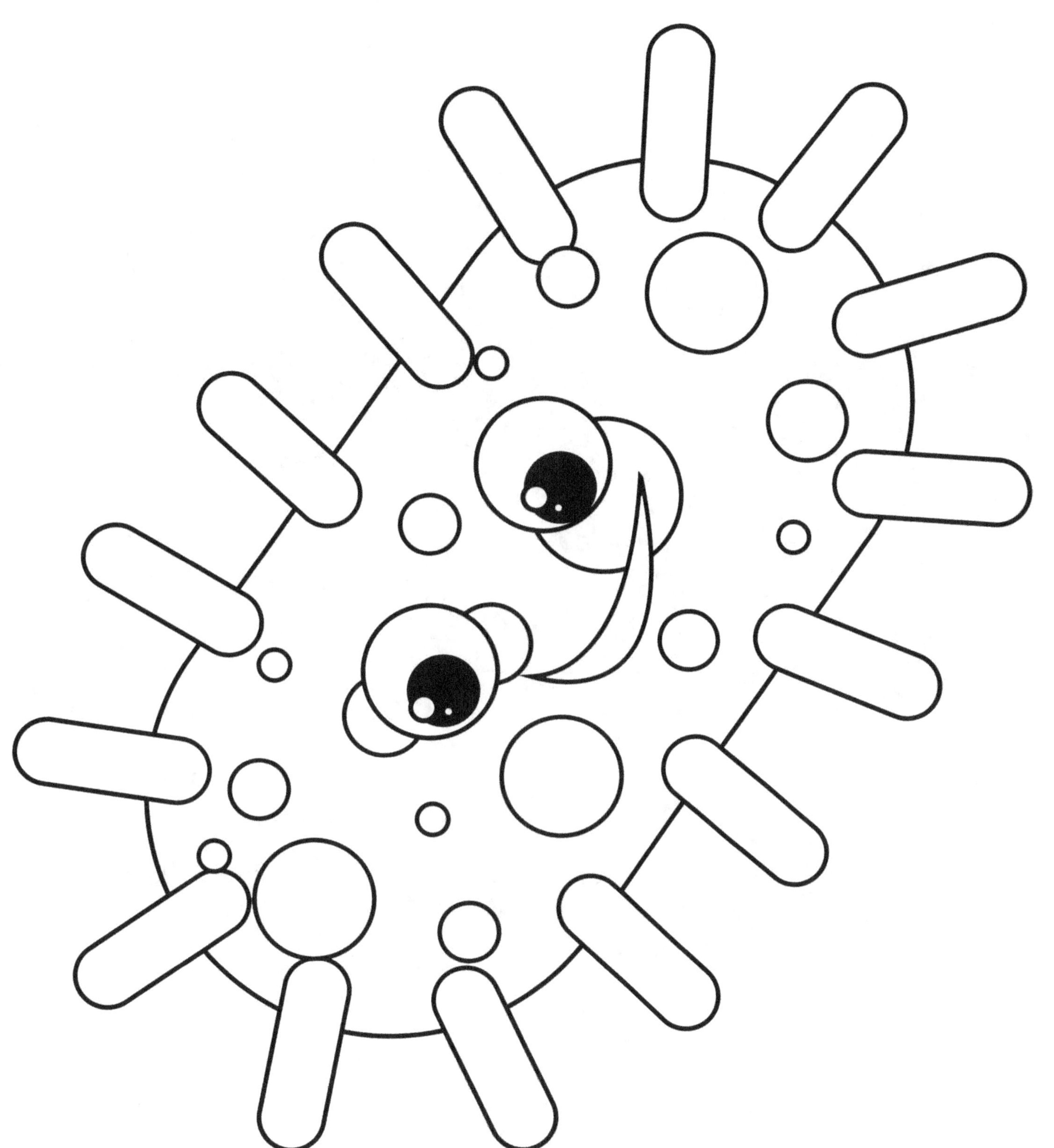

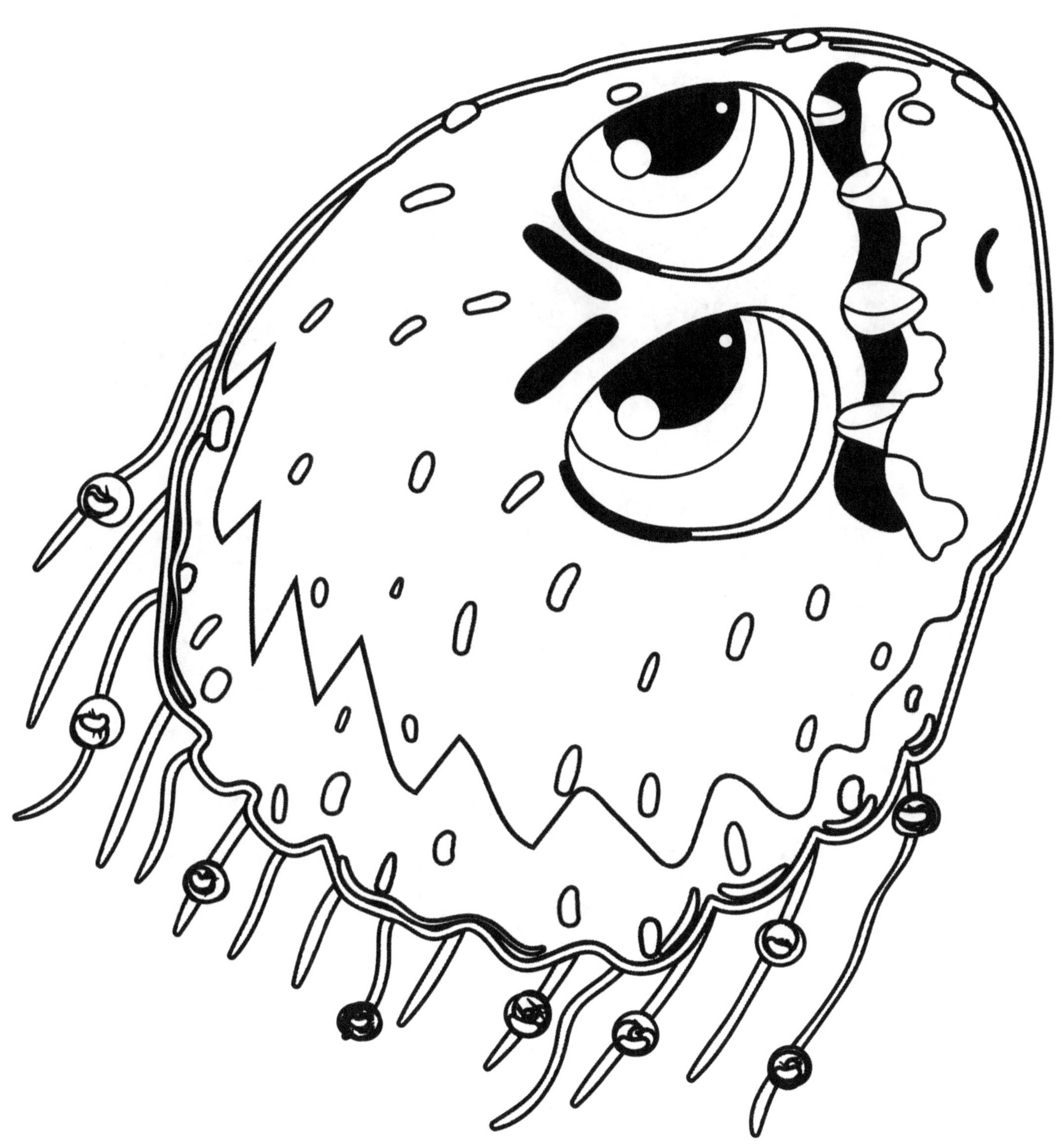

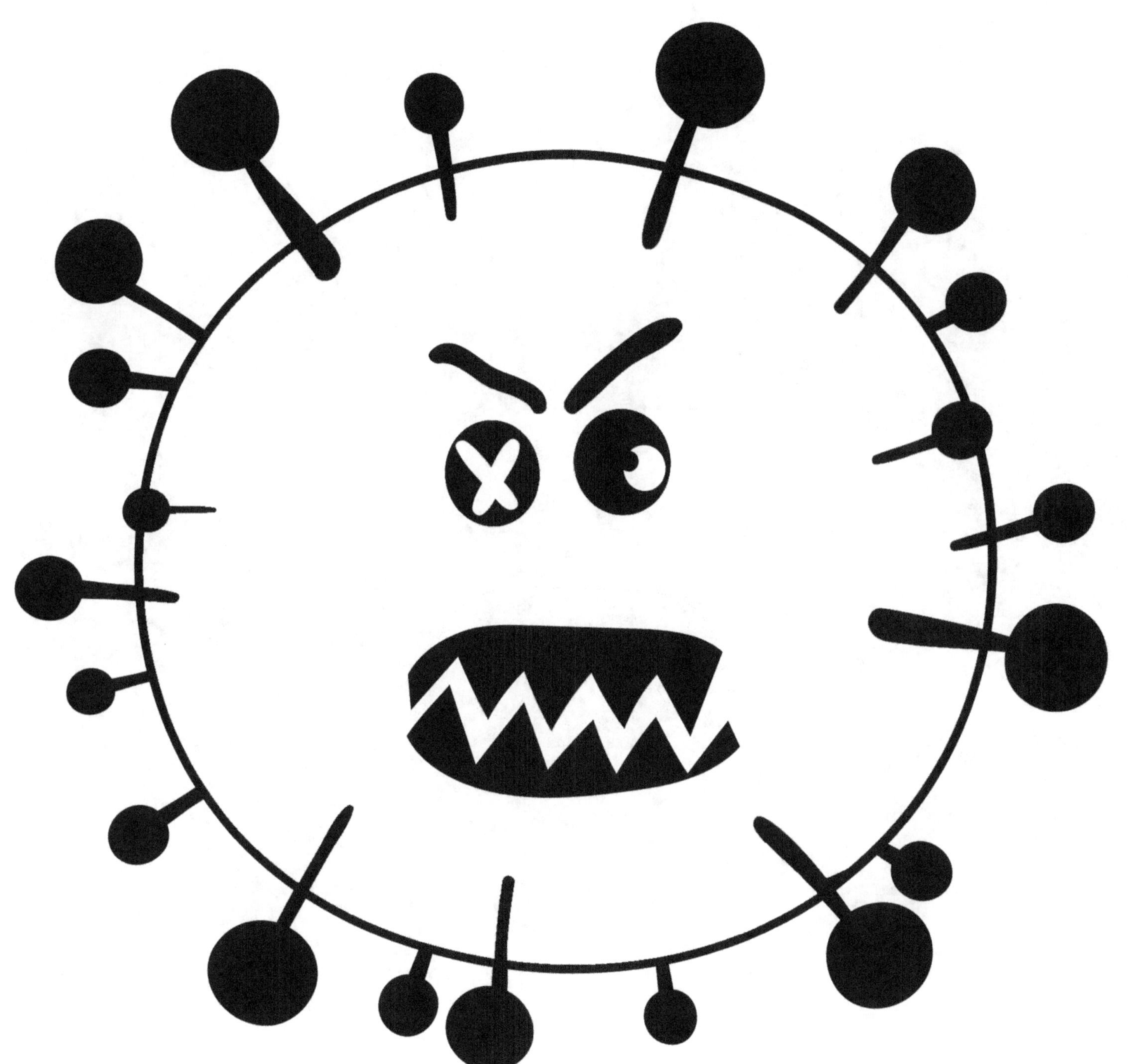

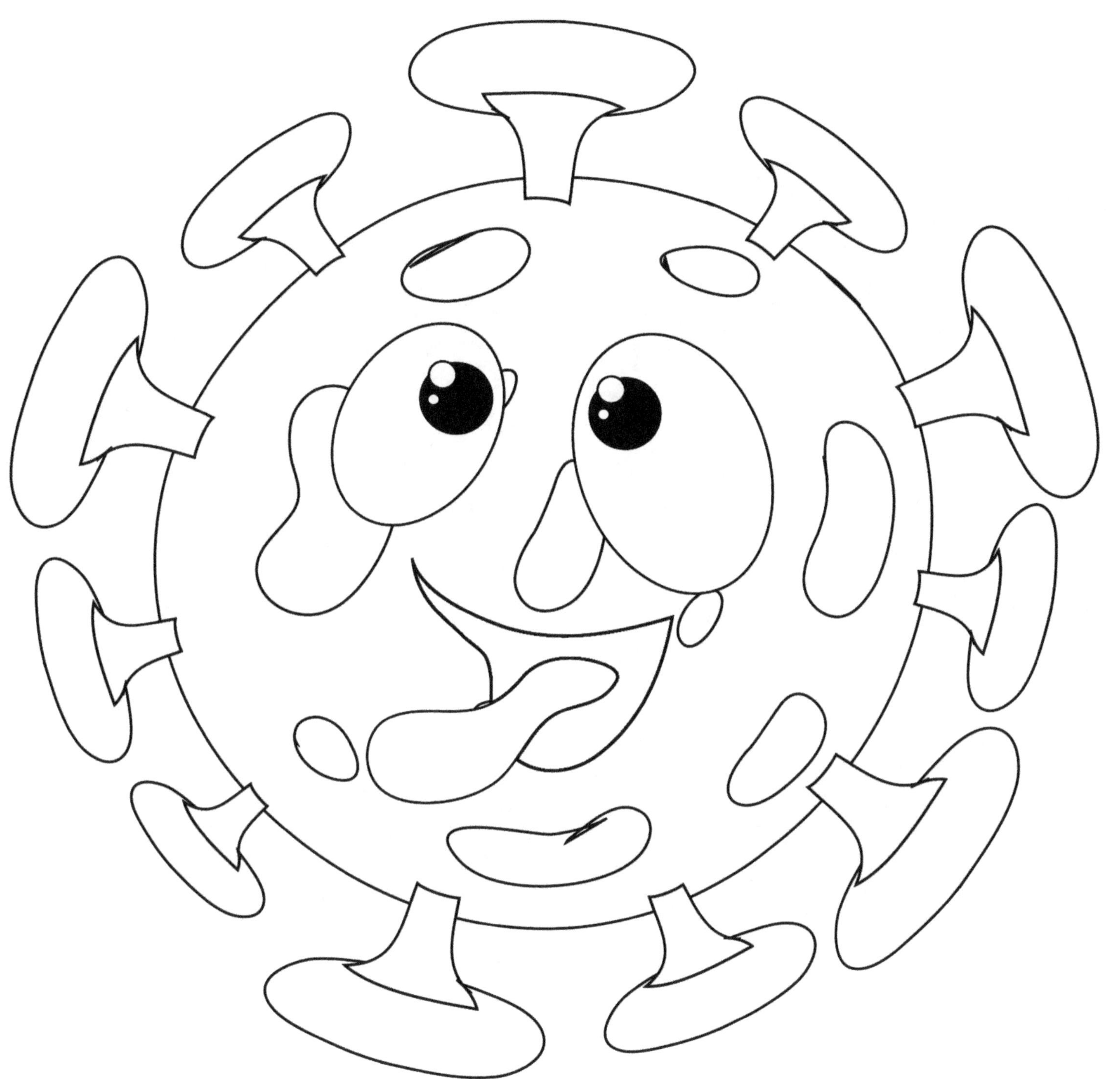

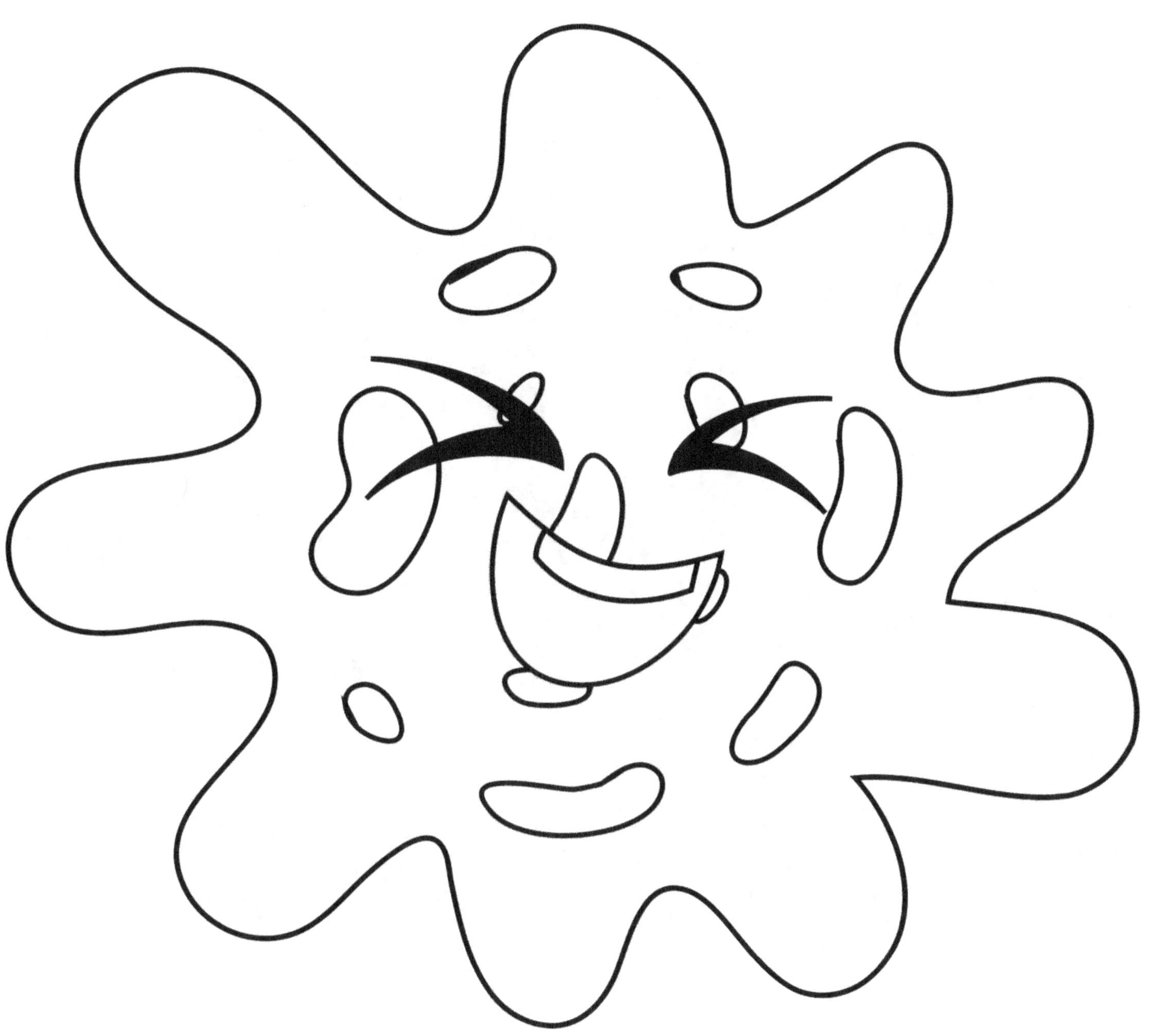

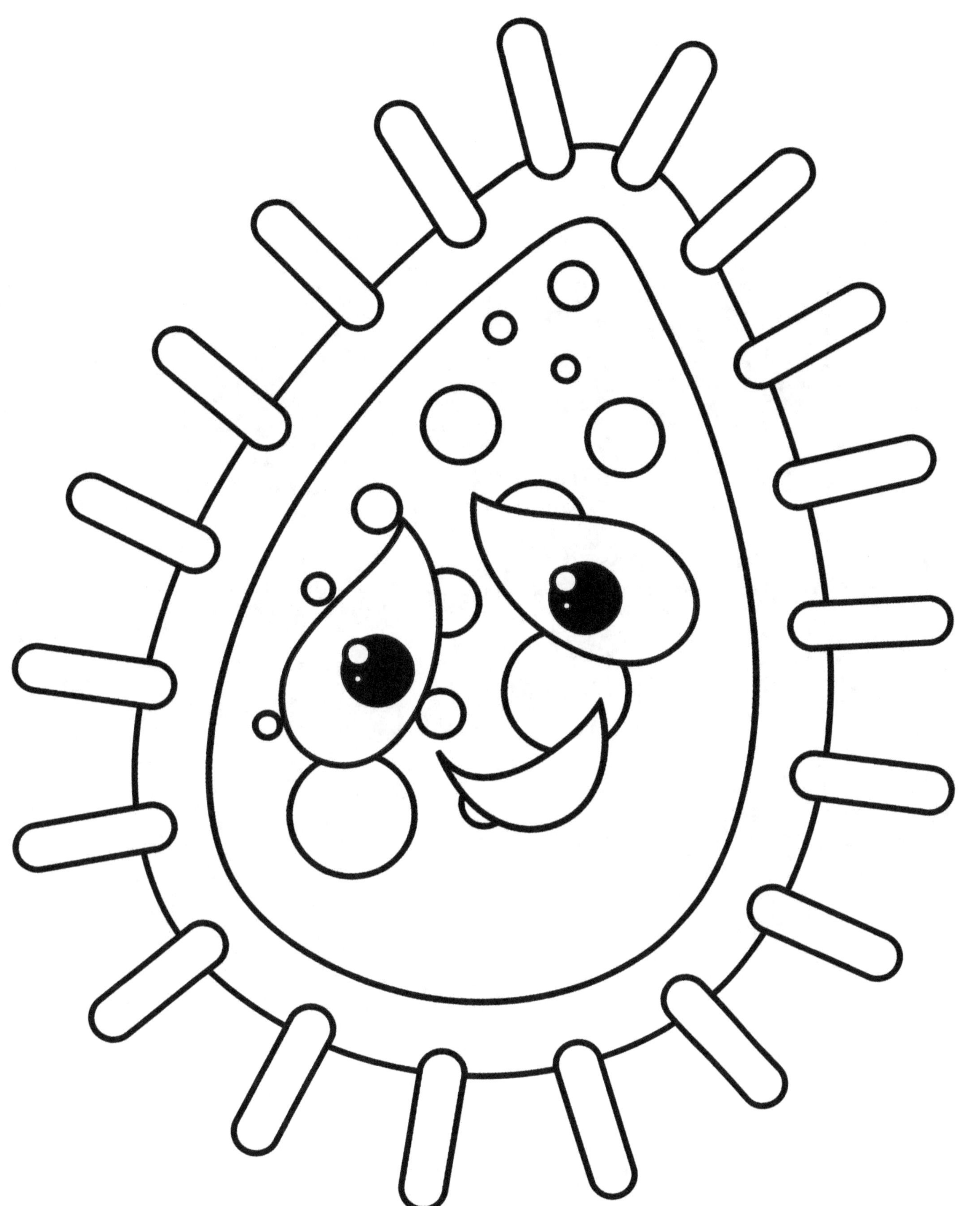

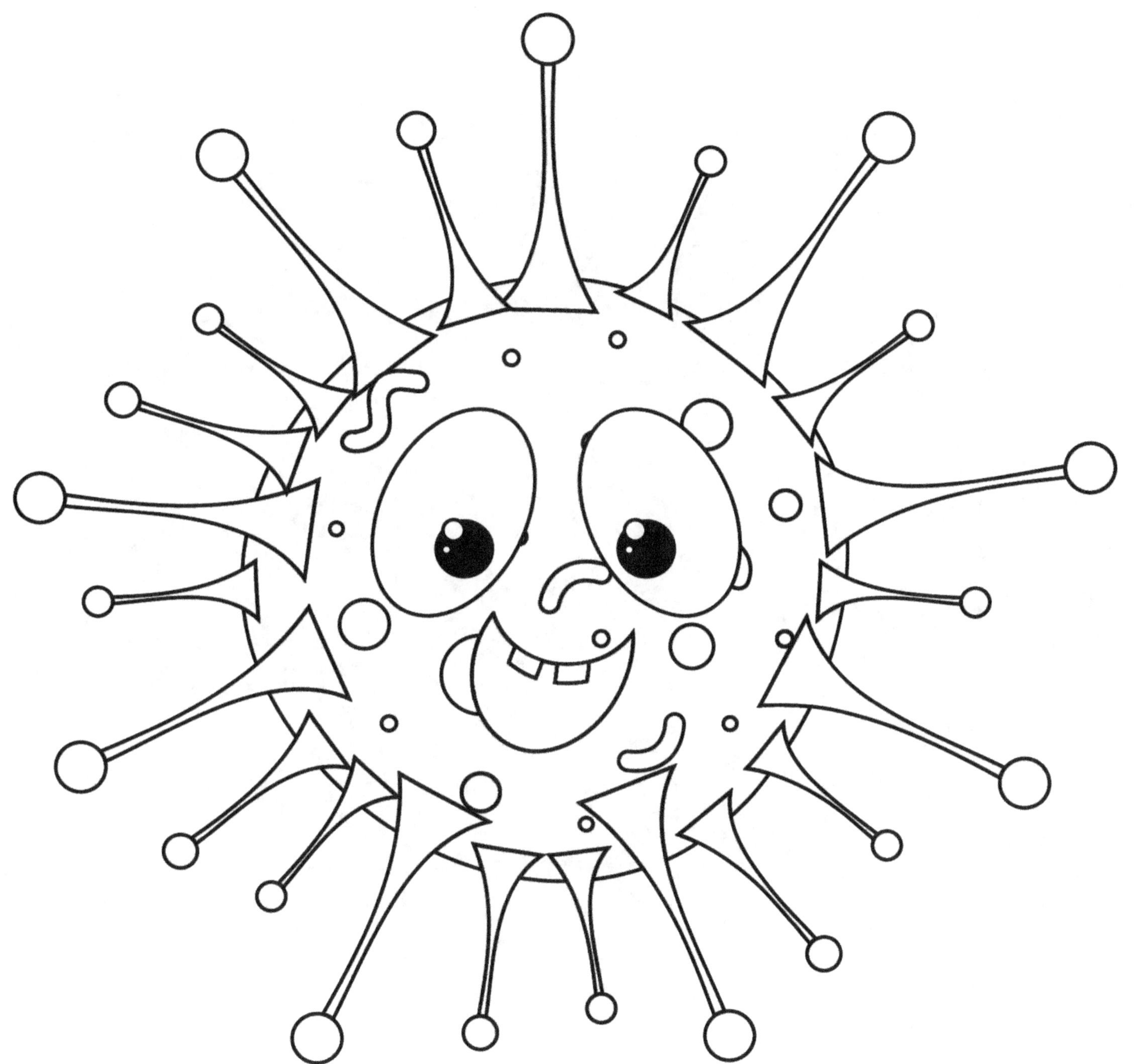

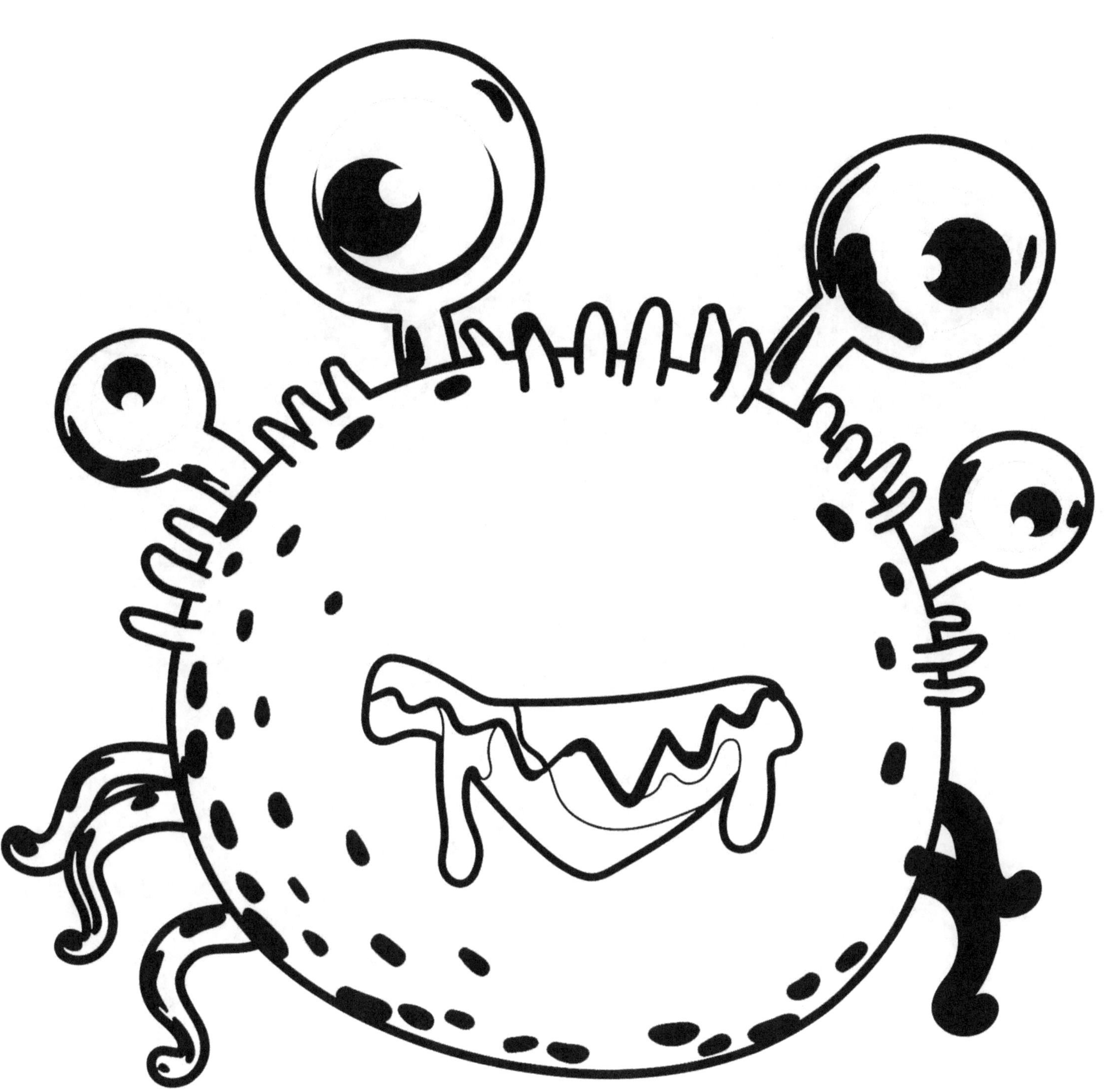

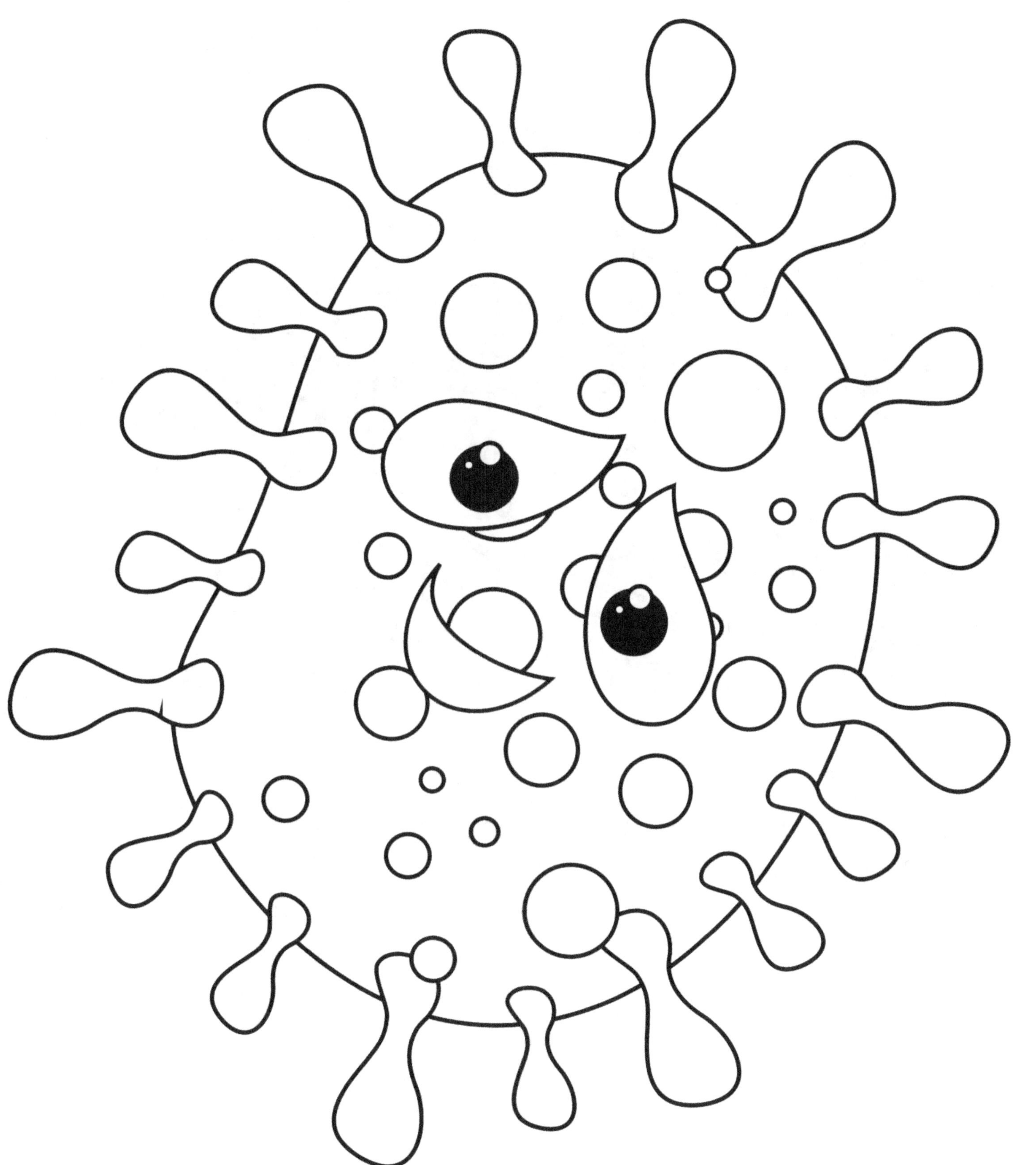

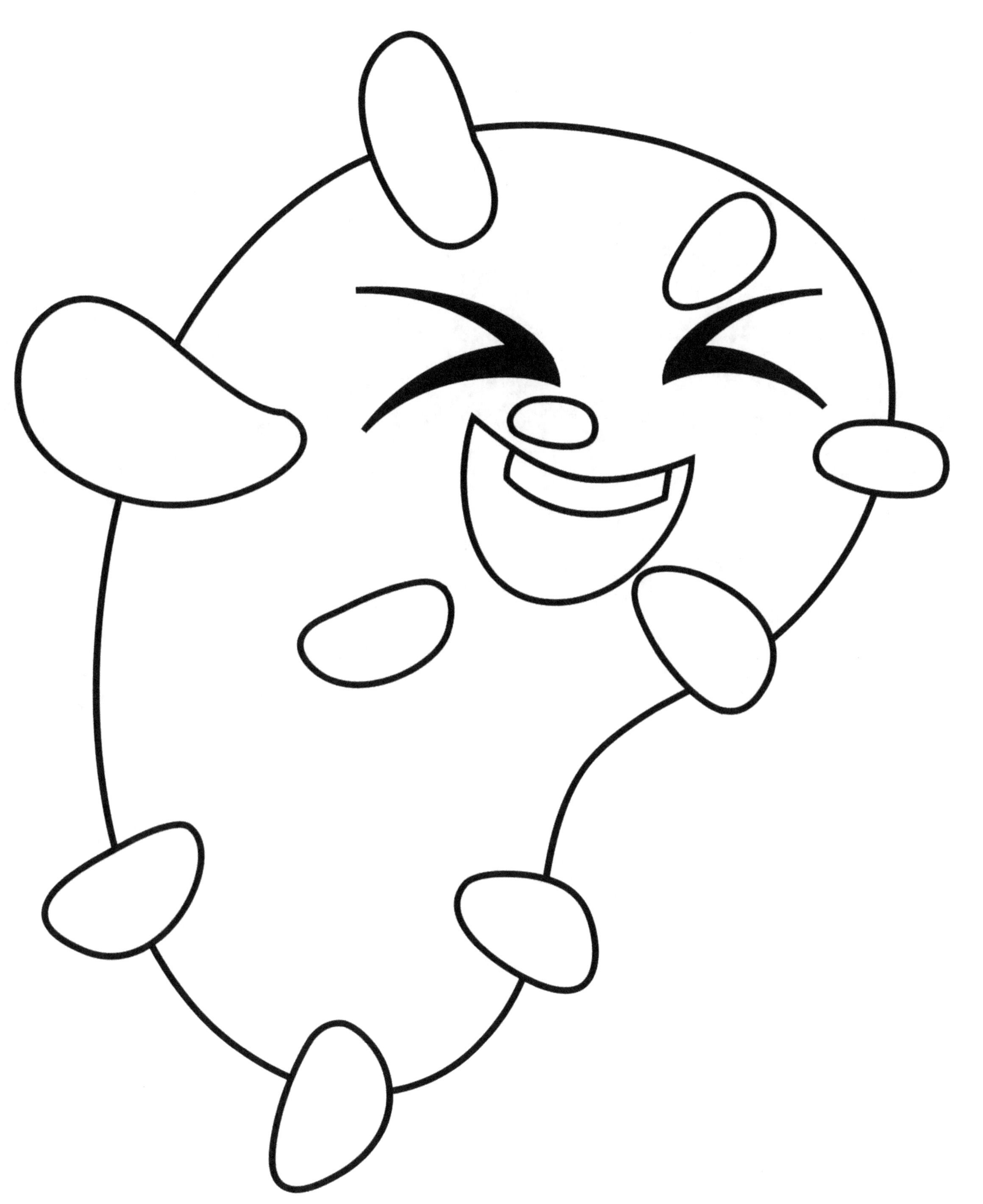

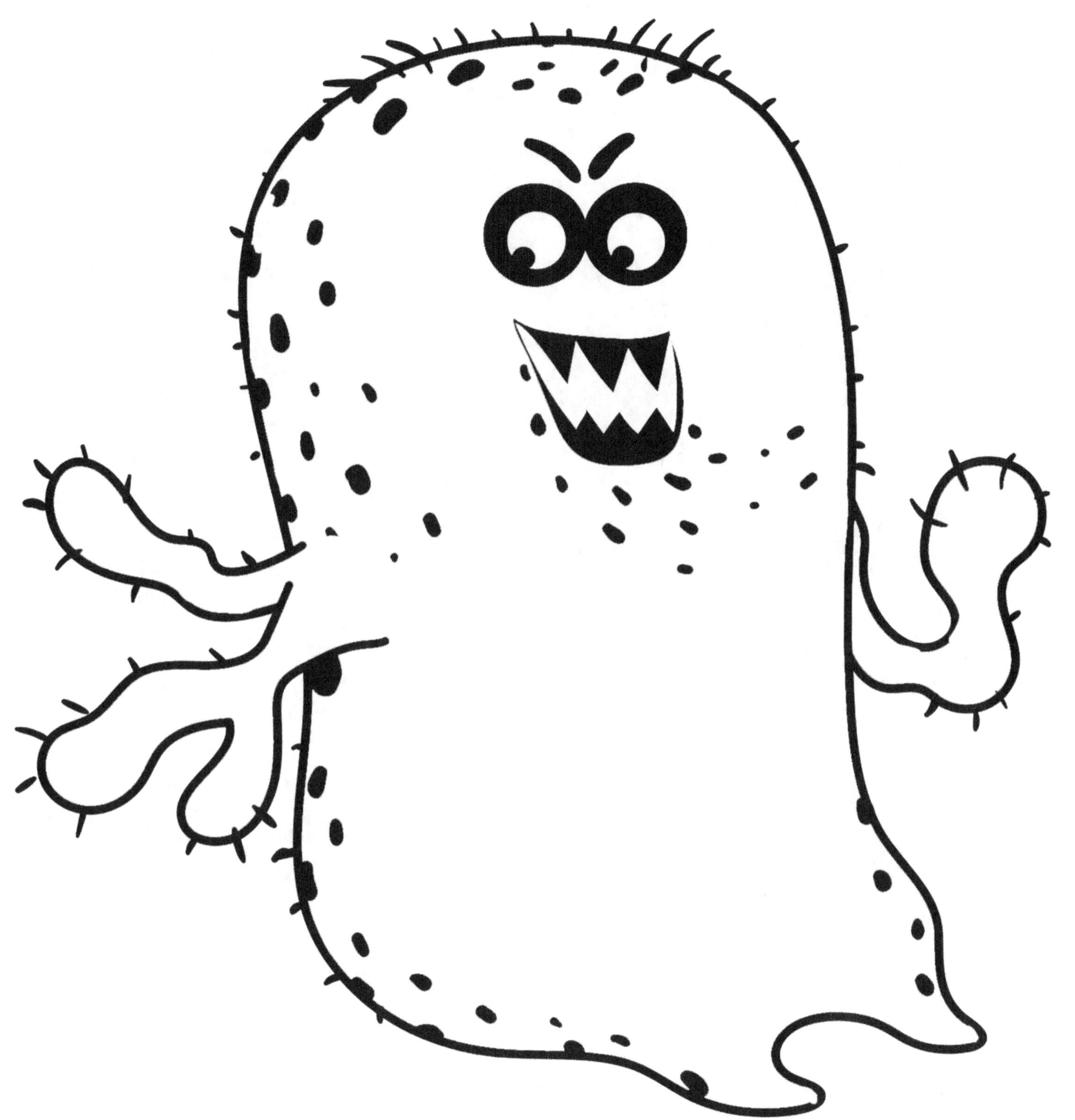

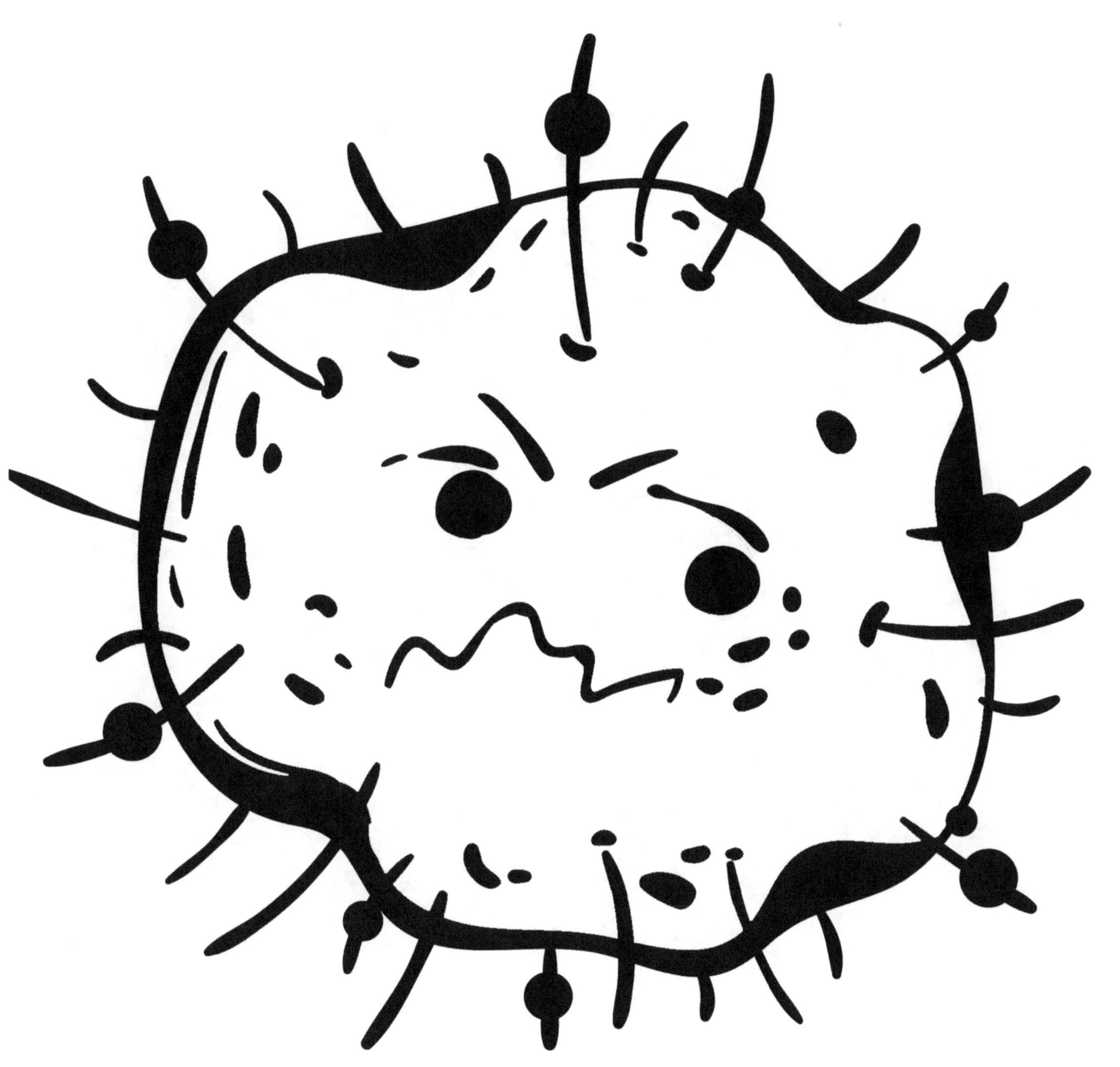

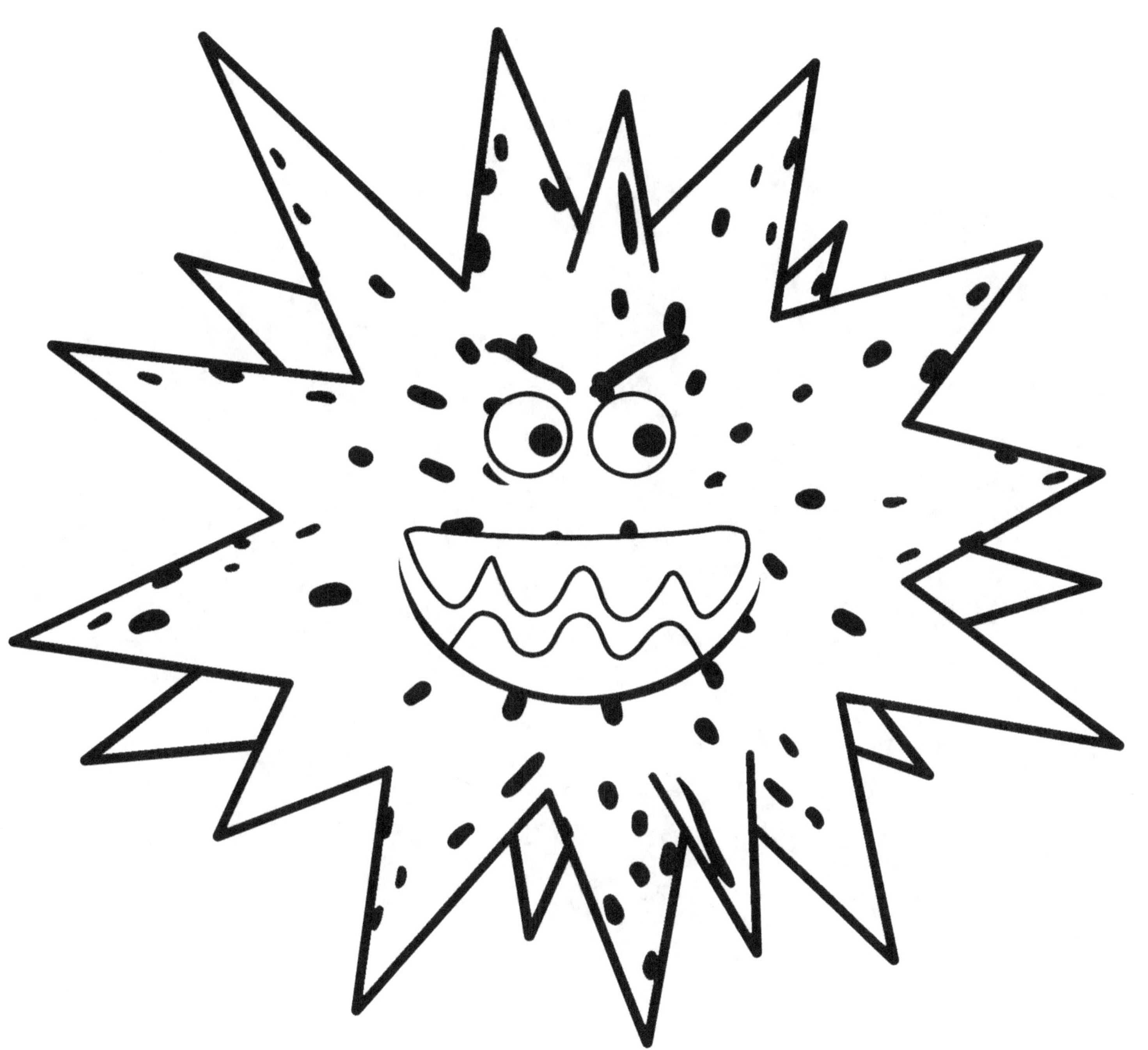

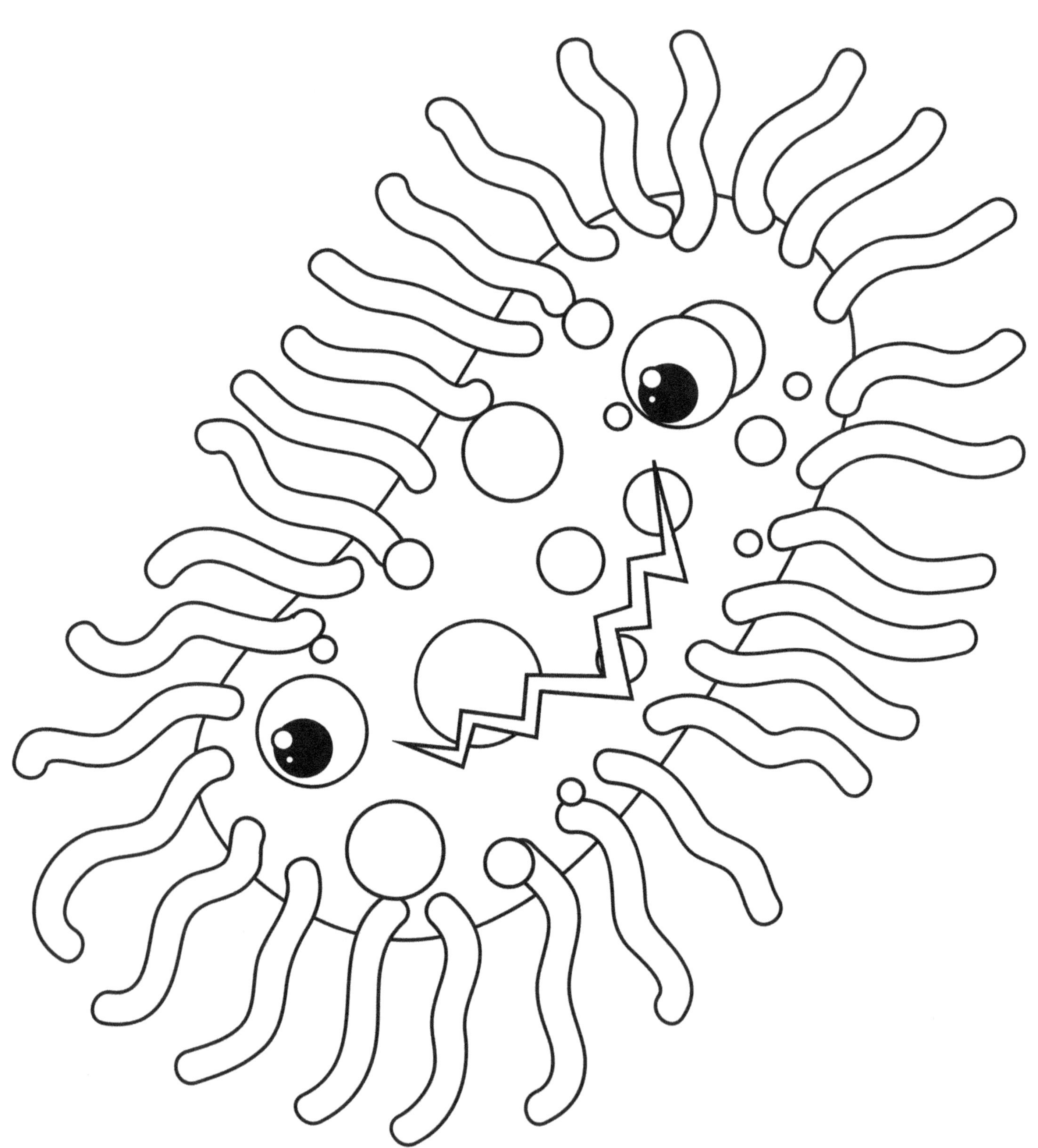

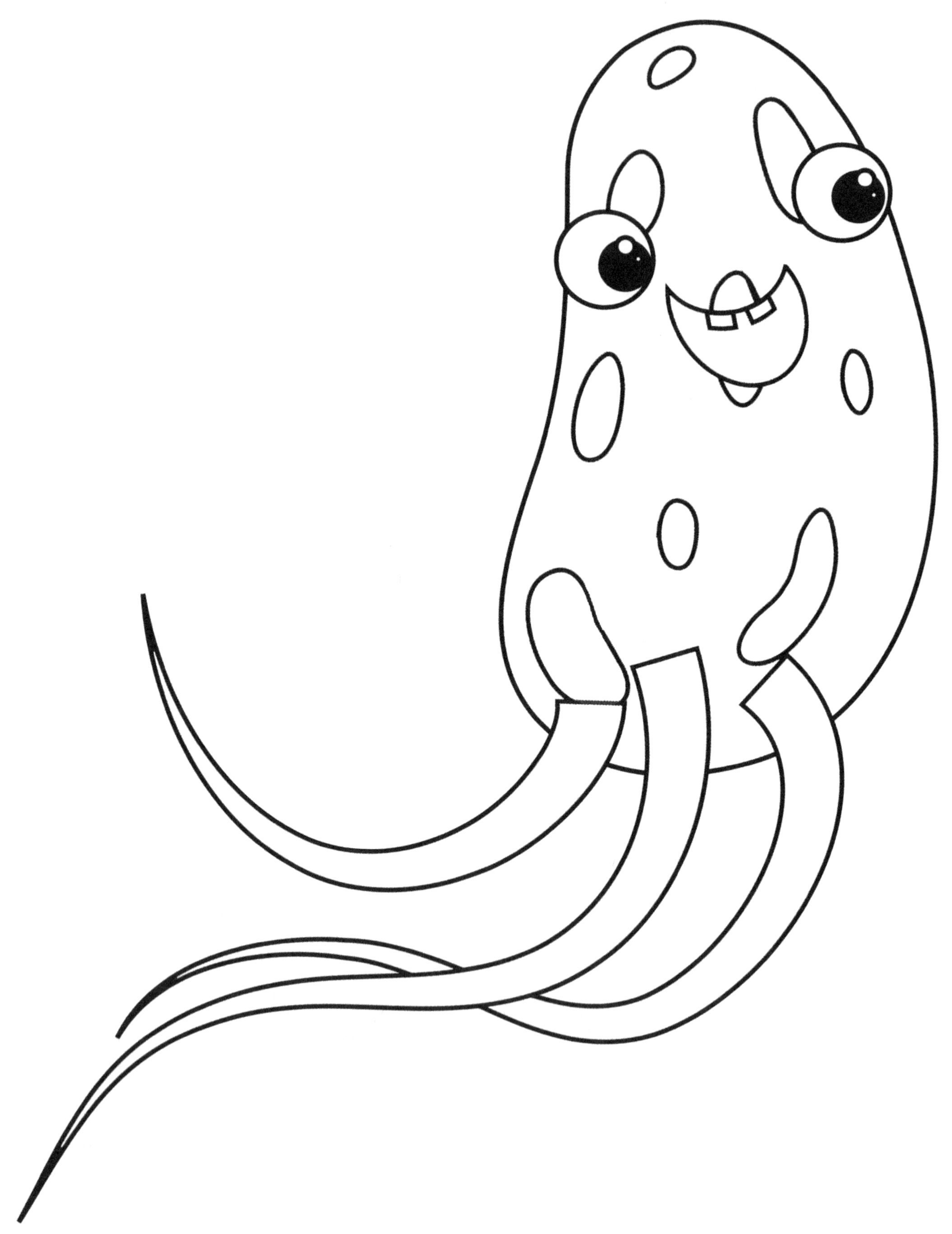